# WHY DOES HE

A Positive Parent's ...
to the Autism Spectrum

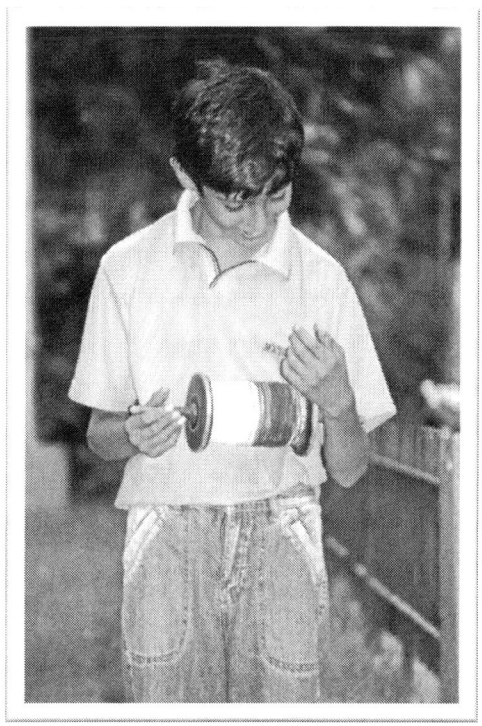

## Stella Waterhouse

Revised edition. Copyright © 2016 by Stella Waterhouse

All rights reserved. No part of this publication may be reproduced, distributed, or transmitted in any form or by any means, including photocopying, recording, or other electronic or mechanical methods, without the prior written permission of the author, except in the case of brief quotations embodied in critical reviews and certain other noncommercial uses permitted by copyright law.

For permission requests, please write to the author, addressed "Attention: Permissions" at stellawaterhouse3@gmail.com

Illustrations by Kate Vargues

*** 

**OTHER BOOKS**

The Positive Approaches Series
*Autism Basecamp: A Toolkit for Positive Parents*
*The Problem is Understanding: A Positive Teacher's Guide to the Autism Spectrum*
*Whoops! A Positive Teacher's Guide to Dyspraxi*a

Autism Decoded Series.
*Book One - The Cracks in the Code*
*Book Two – The Ciphers*
*Book Three – The Source Code*
*Book Four – Decryption*

**Download your FREE Gift from:**
**www.gerrysorrillpublishers.com**

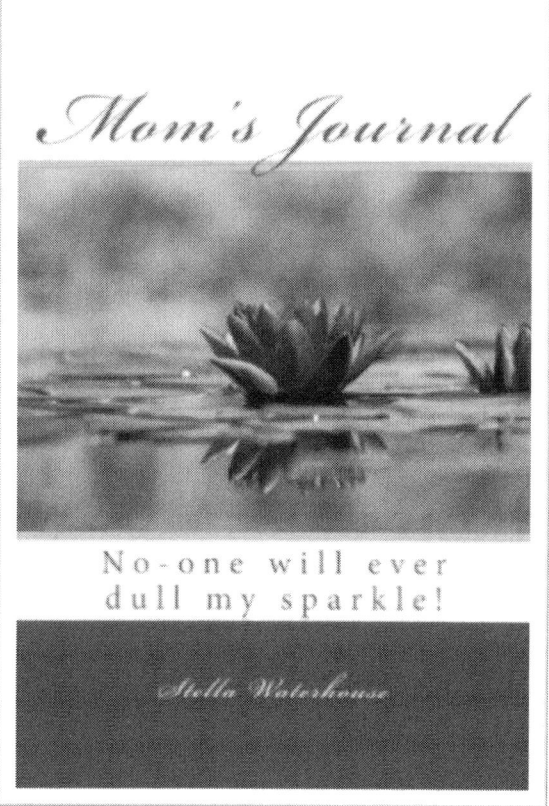

## Other FREEBIES re AUTISM

**Here are some FREE tools to help you on your journey.**

Grab the FREE checklist to help you identify whether your child has visual differences.

Have a child with auditory difficulties? Want to help? Get your FREE mini-course about the Auditory Differences and the Soundsrite Program.

Claim your FREE *Dietary Diary* here

Claim your FREE copy of *The Food Detectives Guide* here

Go to: www.autismdecoded.com or use the QR code

\*\*\*

**CONTENTS**

| | |
|---|---|
| INTRODUCTION | Page 7 |
| | |
| A PARENT'S GUIDE | 9 |
| Criteria | |
| Understanding | 12 |
| From Child to Adolescent | 13 |
| | |
| GROWING UP | 15 |
| Emotions | |
| Exposure Anxiety | 17 |
| Understanding | 18 |
| Thought | 19 |
| The Effects of Visual Thinking in ASD | 20 |
| Physical Development | 21 |
| | |
| THROUGH THE LOOKING GLASS . . . | 23 |
| A Visible Difference | 24 |
| Emotional "blindness" | 28 |
| The Princess and The Pea | 29 |
| Nose Pollution | 30 |
| The Torment of Sound | 31 |
| Try It Yourself | 32 |
| | |
| PRIMARY EFFECTS | 36 |
| Anxiety | |
| Other Effects | |
| Coping Strategies | 38 |

| | |
|---|---|
| E-FFECTS NOT DE-FECTS | 41 |
| Learning Differences | |
| Vulnerability | 44 |
| Signs of Bullying | 45 |
| Communication | |
| Cyberbullying | |
| | |
| FOOD FOR THOUGHT | 46 |
| | |
| PARENT POWER | 48 |
| | |
| BOOKS | 50 |
| | |
| FREE GIFT | 51 |

***

## INTRODUCTION

People with Autistic Spectrum Disorders (ASD) often feel they inhabit another planet, which is why some refer to themselves as aliens. Certainly, judging by their reactions, they find this world both impenetrable and frightening.

Such feelings are often thought to result from the difficulties they have in relating to those around them, and their inability - regardless of intellect - to empathize with or communicate their emotions to others, in the way that most people do.

This idea is constantly reinforced by the criteria used in diagnosis which focus mainly upon the difficulties with social relationships and communication. These though are merely the tip of the iceberg.

Since autism and Asperger's syndrome were identified in the 1940s many articles and books have been written by or featured people who are living with autism or Asperger's syndrome. Such accounts have come, over several decades, from people of various ages and abilities living in different parts of the globe and yet despite this they remain remarkably consistent. Most noticeable is the fact that time and time again one reads or hears the words "fear, terror or confusion" as well as accounts of abnormal sensory experiences.

These comments are supported by those people with autism or Asperger's syndrome who are able to talk about their experiences.

The accounts of abnormal sensory experiences have been given further credence over the years by Dr Bernard Rimland and Dr Carl Delacato and since then, by the well-researched and documented work of those who study neuro-developmental delay. Indeed, similar (but less severe) abnormal sensory perceptions exist amongst many other groups of people: from those with physical problems like migraine to those with learning disabilities such as dyslexia, dyspraxia or attention problems.

This book aims to give a brief overview of the problems faced by children with ASD. Information on the better known aspects of these conditions has been kept relatively brief so that more space can be given to those lesser known but vitally important aspects: that of the sensory problems and anxiety for, as you will see, many of the child's apparently odd mannerisms or bizarre behaviors can be explained by their relationship to either the sensory problems or to anxiety. Thus taking an extra-large step over a threshold may indicate visual problems, whilst compulsive or obsessive or compulsive actions relate to anxiety.

While the text refers to "the child" or "children" these problems certainly affect both adolescents and adults too. Ageing does not necessarily mean that the problems or their effects diminish in intensity - although many people do find ways to compensate for or cope with the problems.

***

## A PARENT'S GUIDE.

Both autism and Asperger's syndrome affect more boys than girls but there are several differences between the two conditions; as is now being confirmed by the latest research using brain scans.

Even so in the mid-2013 the American Psychiatric Association published the fifth edition of the Diagnostic and Statistical Manual of Mental Disorders (DSM-5) in which the criteria for ASD were modified to exclude the diagnoses of Asperger Syndrome, Pervasive Developmental Disorder Not Otherwise Specified or Disintegrative Disorder.

While the diagnosis now given is simply termed Autistic Spectrum Disorder many of those formerly diagnosed with Asperger's syndrome continue to think of themselves in that way.

**Criteria**

Although symptoms must begin in early childhood, when mild they are often may not be recognized fully until the child begins school or even later. Thus the new criteria are based on functional impairment, currently or historically, in two main areas:

1) Social communication/interaction. Examples include:

- Problems reciprocating social or emotional interaction, including difficulty establishing or maintaining back-and-forth

conversations and interactions, inability to initiate an interaction, and problems with shared attention or sharing of emotions and interests with others.
- Severe problems maintaining relationships — ranges from lack of interest in other people to difficulties in pretend play and engaging in age-appropriate social activities, and problems adjusting to different social expectations.
- Nonverbal communication problems such as abnormal eye contact, posture, facial expressions, tone of voice and gestures, and an inability to understand these.

2) Restricted and repetitive behaviors (at least two of which need to be present). These include:

- Stereotyped or repetitive speech, motor movements or use of objects.
- Excessive adherence to routines, ritualized patters of verbal or non-verbal behavior, or excessive resistance to change.
- Highly restricted interests that are abnormal in intensity or focus.
- Hyper/hypo reactivity to sensory input or unusual interest in sensory aspects of the environment.

Prior to this change in the criteria it was considered that those with Asperger's syndrome shared the problems of social interaction and had repetitive behaviors or obsessive traits. However, they were thought to differ from children with autism because they had no significant delay in the development of language or in their cognitive and self-help skills or in their curiosity about the environment.

Asperger's syndrome was also generally linked to people of average (or above average) intelligence, many of whom cope relatively well with daily life. Even so it is important to note that some children with autism have similar abilities too.

Other problems commonly found amongst children on the autistic spectrum include attention problems and/or hyperactivity and dyslexia. In addition, epilepsy affects approximately 1/3 of these children.

The autistic spectrum describes the wide range of functioning and intellectual ability found amongst such children. At one end are those who have severe (and very obvious) learning difficulties, some of whom will remain dependent on others throughout their lives. Such children will often have been diagnosed at an early age and many will have been placed either within a special school or a special needs unit.

Others, with more moderate learning difficulties (who often used to be diagnosed with Asperger's syndrome) may be educated in Speech and Language units although now, with the advent of inclusion, many of the "higher functioning" and more verbal children are likely to be placed within a mainstream school.

At the far end of the spectrum are those ("high functioning") children whose symptoms are much more subtle. They tend to cope relatively well in most situations and may escape diagnosis until much older - if it happens at all. Thus many progress reasonably well at nursery or preschool, although increasing pressures and expectations can make life difficult as they get older. Indeed, for some, regardless of intellect, their apparently odd behaviors prove so bewildering and problematic within the classroom setting that they eventually lead to exclusion. Unfortunately, such Behavioural problems can mask their social inability and may sometimes lead to misdiagnosis or inappropriate treatment. In adult life such people may hold down jobs and have families but will generally be considered odd or eccentric.

A similarly wide spectrum is also found in other spheres:

- Sociability. This ranges from children who totally ignore their peers (although they may seek out adults if they need things), those who make limited contact with other children and yet others who, in contrast, may be overly sociable.

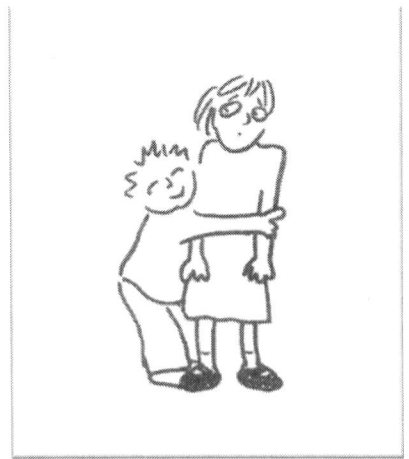

- Speech may be non-existent, consist of echolalia (i.e. repeating whatever is said to them) or simple phrases or alternatively, be extremely clear.

**Understanding.**

All such children (regardless of age, diagnosis, verbal ability or intelligence) have immense difficulties in understanding other people and the world around them the reasons for which will be discussed more fully in the following chapters.
Unsurprisingly such problems make it extremely difficult for the child to relate to other people or make friends. Thus they:

- are unable to "read" facial expressions or body language.
- have difficulties in relating to other people and making friends.
- have a limited understanding of other people's feelings and their own.
- may be unable to control their feelings in an age appropriate manner.
- find it difficult to cope with change.

**From Child to Adolescent.**

Each child's ability to cope with and adapt to his problems will be different and may also vary according to other factors such as the situation, his mood or health.

Although there will be some exceptions, as a general rule the younger child will be confused by his problems and these may cause some bizarre or erratic reactions.

In contrast the older child will have developed various coping strategies which may make him less prone to Behavioural problems. Unfortunately, this can often lead to greater withdrawal thereby inhibiting his ability to learn.

The natural turbulence of adolescence is often compounded by the lack of awareness and the continuing problems of literalness and can give rise to some "strange" confusions - as with the 14-year-old who, being totally unaware that he was growing taller, became very distressed "because the adults around him were shrinking."

Generally, people are much more tolerant of bizarre or difficulties behaviors in the younger child than they will be of the adolescent whose behavior seems apparently "infantile" or beyond control.

While this makes it extremely important for the child to learn that certain behaviors are unacceptable in social situations great care is needed. It is pointless to expect compliance (to the norm) if the child is unable to understand what is being asked of him or if the situation makes your demands totally unrealistic.

It is vital therefore that, before developing unrealistic expectations or making demands on the child, both parents and professionals learn to understand exactly why the child behaves as he does in certain situations.

***

## GROWING UP

Simplistically, every aspect of development, from the emotional to the physical, is like a series of building blocks placed one upon the other. Each has to be placed in just the right position for the structure to be solid. Successful development is only achieved if each stage is completed correctly. If any stage is either missing or incomplete the child's progress can be damaged or slowed (as it often is in autism and Asperger's syndrome) and that can have far reaching consequences.

### Emotions

All too often the person with ASD appears "emotionally immature." This is because the onset of ASD, for whatever reason, disrupts the development of self-awareness. It also curtails the child's ability to interact with other people – that vital process which helps each child learn to understand his feelings, deal with them appropriately and develop self-control and empathy.

Although this does not necessarily apply to all children those affected can have any one (or several) of the following problems:

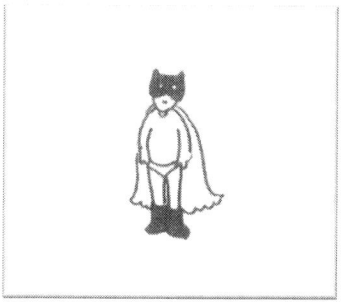

- have little or no "sense of self."
- "hides himself" by copying the actions, speech and

mannerisms of people he knows or of a character(s) that he has seen on television.
- seem very aloof and independent; looks after himself and shuts other people out.
- have difficulty understanding his feelings - may be overwhelmed by them.
- be unable to cope with his feelings in an age appropriate manner - i.e. his limited or poor self-control means he continues to act like a "terrible two" even when older.
- not necessarily distinguish between your feelings and his own so he will be anxious, sad, happy, etc. whenever you are.
- have difficulty relating to parents and/or peers appropriately.
- lack empathy - has little or limited understanding of other people's feelings.

Even so some children do eventually develop some degree of self-awareness, self-control and empathy.

Meanwhile others retain the infant's ability to sense things and remain acutely attuned to other people's feelings; which they may act out at times.

Such awareness can also give rise to a "need" to please other people which can have unexpected consequences so that whilst children with ASD do not generally lie they may sometimes give the answer they "feel" is wanted rather than the correct one.

**Exposure Anxiety**

Many of children also suffer from Exposure Anxiety. This condition, identified by Donna Williams in her book of the same name, can be quite crippling. Although the roots of this problem are complex basically it is similar to feeling acutely self-conscious.

Children like this find any attention from other people as potentially threatening. Thus they feel "exposed" each time another person looks at them, talks to them or even compliments them. This has several different effects as the child may:

- feel unable to do things for himself if other people are around. Thus he: may use other people to carry out tasks for him - such as using another person's hand to turn a door handle, picking something up etc.
- will only do things/help himself/sing when he feels unobserved
- avoid using personal pronouns
- have various speech "differences" which can mean that speech is: nonexistent; used only when he feels unobserved; limited to a few "safe" words or phrases or very repetitive.

In order to cope with exposure anxiety, the child may attempt to "block out" the triggers. This can lead to some strange reactions as he may ignore the people he likes most or respond to direct praise by losing interest, disowning (or even destroying) his achievements.

**Understanding.**

His ability to socialize, explore and play will also be curtailed by the onset of the problems and this, in turn, will affect the development of his cognitive skills and understanding. All too often this can leave his level of understanding out of kilter with his intelligence in some areas. This can mean that he may:

- not understand apparently simple concepts. One example of this is the ability to know that a dining chair, an armchair and a picture of a chair all have something in common.
- not necessarily take something which has been learnt in one context and apply it in another situation.
- have difficulty understanding abstract concepts.
- take things literally.

Taking things literally can cause confusion and distress. Thus he may get upset by words or phrases which have more than one meaning: like the child who got had a tantrum when offered "marble" cake.

Other things that are hard to understand include: sarcasm; double meanings (as in many jokes); idioms such as "on second thoughts" as well as the increasing tendency to use verbs as nouns - e.g. "that film was a good watch" or "the game is a must see."

**Thought.**

While the pre-verbal infant thinks in pictures most adults think in different ways in different situations: thinking in words when they are reading and in pictures if they are designing a garden or a house.

The majority of people think in words at the same speed as speech and thus they "hear" what they are reading in their minds. In contrast many people with dyslexia think in pictures instead – something which also applies to some – but not all – people on the autistic spectrum.

The work in this area was initiated by Ron Davis. He had many problems throughout his child-hood, but the one he found most daunting was his inability to learn to read. Despite that Mr. Davis became an extremely successful engineer and eventually made a fortune. Finally, after managing to teach himself to read and write he decided to try to help other people overcome this problem too and founded the Davis Dyslexia Association International (DDAI).

The DDAI consider that thinking in pictures becomes a major hindrance when people learn to read. This is because the person who thinks in pictures builds up a picture in his mind, adding to it as more concepts arise which is far faster than thinking in words and can make the person very good at many subjects such as the arts or computing.

Unfortunately, though it places the child at a real disadvantage when he learns to read. This is because while it is easy to visualize nouns, verbs and some other words other words (particularly abstract concepts such as pronouns or adverbs) like "I, you, it, with, if", or "and" are much harder to visualize. Thus the sentence "His house is big and it has a chimney pot" would seem to read " … house… big … … … chimney pot." Confusing! Does the word big relate to the house or simply the chimney pot?

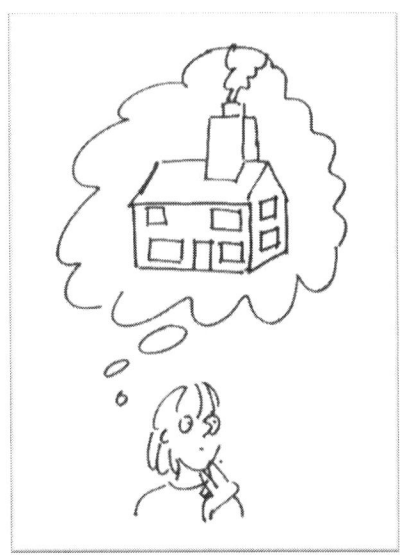

**The effects of visual thinking in ASD.**

Some people with ASD are visual thinkers too. One of the most well-known is Dr Temple Grandin. Despite having Asperger's syndrome, she gained a doctorate in animal sciences and now designs equipment for handling cattle which is used in many of the cattle stations in America. As her book Thinking in Pictures shows, this ability has been of great help to her in conceiving and developing her designs.

It is probable that visual thinking could also underlie some of the cognitive problems and speech difficulties that people with ASD have.

If you cannot easily conceive the meaning of such words, how can you possibly understand what people are saying to you - or respond easily and fluently? There is a time-lapse as you "translate" the words into an informative picture and then "translate" back into the words that you need to respond with. No wonder such children find it hard to "keep up" with the conversation.

**Physical Development**

Many children on the autistic spectrum have a degree of Neuro-developmental delay (NDD). This leaves the whole system with a minor flaw like a tiny crack in the foundations of a building the results of which are often not be apparent until much later.

Although the initial problems can easily be missed, if the problems begin in infancy the baby could be unusually irritable; difficult to feed and/or a poor sleeper. Alternatively, he may seem exceptionally placid or simply be slow to reach the "normal" developmental milestones. In contrast others will develop in an apparently "normal" manner until later when that tiny flaw causes a problem. This can mean that one stage of development is either shorter than "normal" or missed out completely, as with the child who "bottom shuffles" and then walks without crawling or creeping in between. This itself creates further problems as all these stages are necessary if the visual system, hand-eye coordination and praxis are to develop correctly.

Thus NDD gives rise to a wide range of problems the most debilitating of which are the Sensory Problems which generally affect all the senses - albeit to varying degrees. With the exception of vision, which is more complex, the effects fall into three groups as Dr Carl Delacato discovered in the 1970s. Thus the child may be hyper (over) sensitive, hypo (under) sensitive or alternatively, a mixture of both.

Many such children have physical problems too, which can include difficulties with any or all of the following:

- Movement, balance and vision. These are all controlled by the vestibular system - which is located within the inner ear.
- Praxis - the ability to plan and/or carry out actions. Thus some children will have a degree of dyspraxia and might also have associated problems with perception, thought or speech.
- Sensory Integration - the way we organize and makes sense of the information that the body receives from the senses.

\*\*\*

## THROUGH THE LOOKING GLASS . . .

Grow up anywhere in the world and, while the language and climate differs, much remains the same. From birth, the majority of us can see our parents and hear their voices. Our senses help us learn about the world. Initially we learn to associate pleasure and comfort with the touch, feel and smell of our mother, from the warmth of her body to the taste of milk.

As we grow we play with our food enjoying its feel as much as its taste and texture. We have fun playing peek-a-boo and other games with our parents, "exploring" our toys and the objects around us with all our senses. When we are hurt we get comfort from our mother's touch and find her voice soothing. In short we use our senses to learn about relationships, the wider world and our place in it.

Imagine though, growing up in a different way, where nothing is quite as it seems. You are not blind but you cannot see properly (although those around you assume you can). Your mother is just a large blob moving towards you; her outstretched arms may even look quite threatening . . . although you can recognize her when she gets close. However careful she is it hurts when she brushes your hair. Things sparkle in the air. They distract and fascinate you. People frighten you for their faces are disjointed and change when they move. Some of them smell overwhelmingly - of toothpaste, perfume, dogs, smoke. Some noises sound really loud and are immensely frightening, like dragons breathing fire . . .

Background noises impinge on you all the time and stop you from hearing properly when people are talking. Your mother's voice is drowned out by the street noise . . .

This is the world inhabited by the child on the autistic spectrum; who experiences the most bizarre sensations. A world in which the only constants are confusion, terror and fear.

***Be quite clear.***

***This is not a world that the majority of us inhabit.***

Time then to look at each aspect of these problems in turn as we step into a different world: the world inhabited by those with autism and Asperger's syndrome.

**A Visible Difference.**

Vision accounts for over 70% of the information we receive about the world which makes it extremely important to learning. Unfortunately, there are a group of visual problems (which are generally not identified in an ordinary eye test) that can affect reading. These problems (known as visual dyslexia or Irlen syndrome) mean that the child, quite literally, does not see what other people see.

The signs of visual dyslexia include a range of focusing anomalies so that the child often cannot use both eyes together; has a "wandering" eye or a squint. He may also have poor visual acuity or photo-phobia which is not a phobia but rather a physical "over-reaction" to glare, brightness or fluorescence that is outside the control of the person concerned.

Such anomalies can cause a wide range of symptoms. These are individual but when mild include eye-strain; headaches/migraine or clumsiness.

Moderate problems are associated with reading and writing difficulties although these can often be overcome, particularly in the early years when books have large, well-spaced, print. Unfortunately, though, as the child progresses through school, the print and the spaces between lines decrease in size increasing the chance of strange visual effects.

To get some idea of the problems such children have you might want to try reading this page under a <u>very</u> bright light (perhaps by shining a torch on part of it) or by wearing sunglasses as you read. Alternatively, if you need glasses for reading just try it without. Not quite the same but it does give you a little taste of the difficulties.

Thus when reading some children find the letters move and jump off the page or suddenly appear as two texts next to each other. Alternatively, the words may become distorted while the spaces may form "rivers" that cut through the text. This often causes them to lose their place or miss a line.

As the spacing between the lines gradually decreases in size and that makes it harder and harder for the person to read it clearly without seeing a variety of visual distortions while doing so.

Different fonts (the type of text) or a different colored text can cause additional problems too.

To get some idea of these problems try reading this book under different lighting conditions. If you normally wear glasses, try reading it without them. Conversely you could read it with sunglasses on in a darkened room or while shining a bright light on to the page. Difficult isn't it?

Ongoing research indicates that it is likely that many children on the autistic spectrum share similar, but much more severe, visual difficulties. This, plus information gained from people with ASD indicates that they may experience a variety of effects that can include:

- problems judging differences in height or width – particularly noticeable when he steps off a curb or over a threshold.
- difficulty following moving objects – so he may not see an approaching car until it is very close.
- double vision; seeing two separate images at the same time.
- a confused perception of space and size - things may seem at times to change size or shape.
- some things may seem magnified – one child saw a hair as if it were a strand of spaghetti – which can lead to a fascination with tiny things and make him good at doing intricate tasks

Some children are only able to focus on one part of the face at a time so that faces may seem distorted or fragmented and all that he sees clearly may be an eye, a mouth or an earring. Any child who sees in this way is actually only partially-sighted. He lives in a world where nothing is quite as it seems, nothing is constant; where other people (and objects) can, at times, appear to be extremely frightening.

For some children though things are much worse for, like Gunilla Gerland who has Asperger's syndrome, they may simply see a blank face, framed perhaps by dark hair or with a hairy growth over part of it.

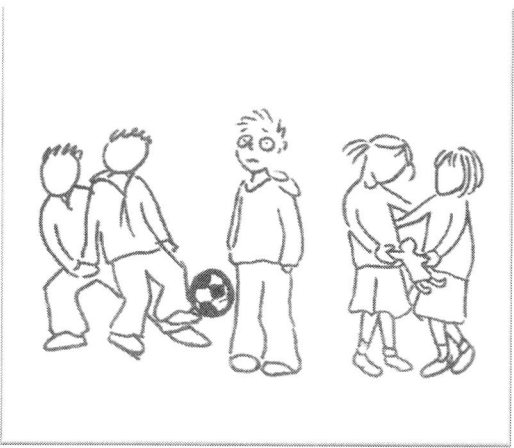

Pictures of faces are stored in a special part of the brain. In some cases, "face blindness" is caused by a malfunction in that part of the brain.

However, there is also a possibility that for some children with ASD this face-blindness actually stems from photo-phobia or poor visual acuity although research has yet to determine the answers.

Certainly if you cannot see correctly the only pictures that you could store would either be blank or extremely bizarre which would make remembering and placing faces almost impossible. Sadly, this can mean that he may not always recognize the important people in his life even if he sees them every day – although as he grows

older he will learn to use other clues such as smell; the way the person's clothes move; or an identifying feature like a mole etc.
**Emotional "blindness."**

Most people communicate their emotions through their facial expressions or their tone of voice as well as words. Children naturally learn how facial expressions and gestures work by watching and interacting with their parents. Face blindness interferes with this process, leaving the child unable to use facial expressions or gestures.

The child with face blindness or other severe visual problems will generally not be able to:

- Identify people correctly by sight alone. Looking at faces close up will give a clearer picture – although he may also use other clues like smell. Thus he may not even recognize you . . .

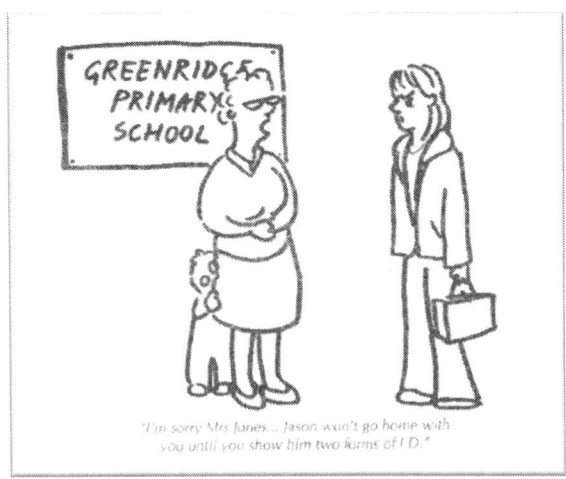

"I'm sorry Mrs Jones...Jason won't go home with you until you show him two forms of I.D."

- Read facial expressions or body language properly - making it impossible for him to communicate or interact with others in a "normal" manner.
- Find his way around an apparently familiar building easily – which can be particularly difficult when in need of a toilet.

Such visual problems cause great anxiety but unfortunately, they frequently remain undiagnosed. Thus both the child and his parents can be unaware that he sees differently from his peers. This compounds the problems and, combined with his inability to cope as others do can lead to frustration and poor self-esteem.

**The Princess and The Pea.**

In the fairy story of that name the princess was unable to sleep because the queen had had a dried pea hidden underneath 20 mattresses. Unfortunately, such sensitivities are not confined to the realm of fantasy.

Sadly, for the "hyper" child normally pleasant stimuli are actually painful and go on and on and on . . . Thus the baby arches away from his mother when she tries to feed him, whilst the toddler moves away to avoid that hug. This child finds a soft, gentle touch more painful than a firm grip and dislikes the feel of the hairbrush, comb or toothbrush.

Some materials will feel irritating or "scratchy" - which is why she may want to wear one particular item of clothing all the time or take her clothes off at every opportunity.

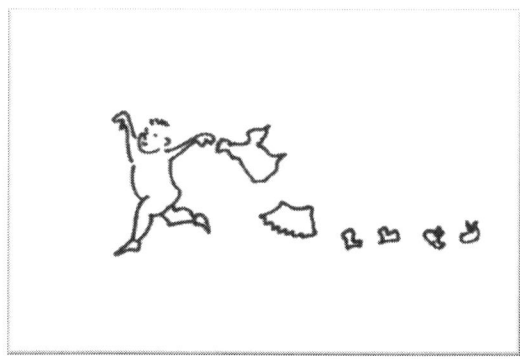

This is a child who probably dislikes finger paints or getting sticky or gritty. Her sensitivity may also extend to the texture of food which may be rejected because it is too lumpy, grainy etc. Confusingly though real pain may either provoke a total over-reaction or be ignored.

Such behaviors are not "autistic" fads. They arise because the child is hypersensitive.

In contrast the hyposensitive child will usually enjoy various vigorous sensations and enjoy physical contact and may even initiate a "rough and tumble." Unfortunately, though he may not always be aware when he hurts or cuts himself.

**Nose Pollution.**

Being "hyper" to smell can have some far-reaching effects. Most of us might find it unpleasant to holiday near a farm where the farmer had been muck-spreading, but after a short time we would "shut the smell out" so that it no longer troubled us. Imagine though if remained aware of it hour after hour . . . Hardly surprising that some everyday smells like disinfectant or perfume lead her to avoid places such as the kitchen or bathroom 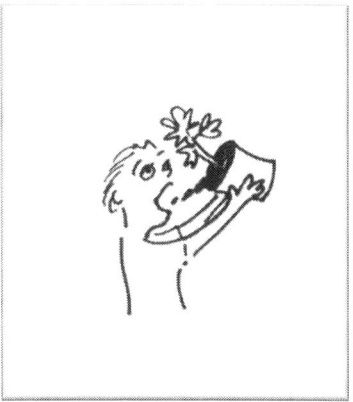 and even some foods. Or that such problems can limit social contact - as with the girl who said that "9 out of 10 people have halitosis."

The relationship between smell and taste may also lead to some food fads. It can also put the "hypo" (under-sensitive) child at risk as his poor sense of smell and resulting lack of awareness may mean that he eats things indiscriminately - whether edible or not.

**The Torment of Sound.**

People generally associate hearing problems with an identifiable hearing loss but there are several other auditory difficulties that can have a devastating effect. These can, at times, make many apparently ordinary situations almost intolerable for the child. The problems include:

- Poor auditory discrimination. He may mishear some letters or words or be unable to pin-point where sound is coming from which can be quite confusing – and makes it seem as if other people are talking nonsense.
- Hyperacusis - hypersensitivity to sound – a condition that also affects some people with tinnitus. This means that he finds some specific everyday sounds painful. The sounds that cause problems are individual and can range from quiet sounds such a clock ticking or people eating to louder sounds like vacuum cleaners and food mixers.
- Loudness intolerance i.e. when the child - cannot tolerate the same level of noise as his peers, so he will get very upset by loud noises such as fire alarms.
- "Supersensitive hearing." He may also be able to hear noises (or conversations) that others are unaware of. (something which can be enhanced by vitamin and mineral deficiencies).
- The majority of children will also be unable to block out background sounds which constantly impinge on them.

**The Effects.**

Many children with ASD are tormented as everyday sounds, that most of us ignore or at least tolerate, constantly impinge and intrude upon them. Such auditory difficulties also:

- make many areas of the home very difficult for him
- make shopping, the playground, classroom and even trips out potentially distressing and frightening.
- can underlie or aggravate speech and language problems.
- mean that child needs to concentrate much harder than his peers in order to make sense of the spoken word – something which can be particularly difficult in noisy situations.

The child with such problems may react to these noises in a variety of ways e.g. blocking his ears; withdrawing into himself; running away from the situation or having a panic attack.

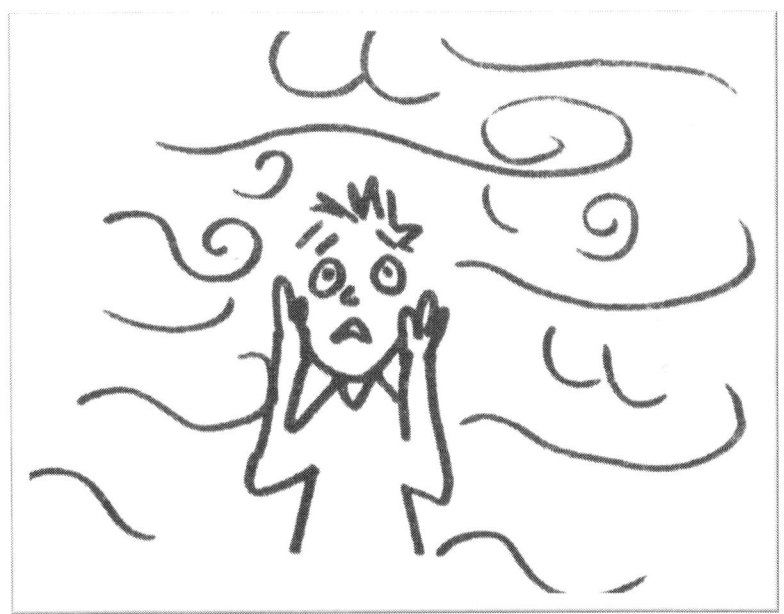

The jumbled information the child receives from his senses causes disorientation and confusion, leaving him in a nightmare world. Worse still, unlike adults who have a wealth of inner experiences to help them survive, the young child simply does not have the resources to cope with such problems.

**Try It Yourself.**

The following passage (adapted from the work of the late Svea Gold who was both an author and therapist) demonstrates just how different and difficult life would be if you were unable to believe your senses.

*Just imagine . . walking your dog on a bright sunny day. While you're walking you prepare a shopping list, write a letter in your mind, and plan your day's work. Now imagine walking the same street, with the same dog, on a dark winter morning in a fog. You can't see more than about thirty feet ahead. The dog will protect you - but it's such a tiny dog! There is a strange noise, to your right. Tap, tap, tap . . . as you get closer, you realize it's just a drainpipe dripping . . . Every sound needs to be analyzed as you go on your way. Suddenly the headlights of a car appear behind you, and as you step to the side, the car slows down and comes to a stop. All the kidnapping shows that you've ever seen on TV seem to turn into reality. The car starts off again, and the paper girl waves*

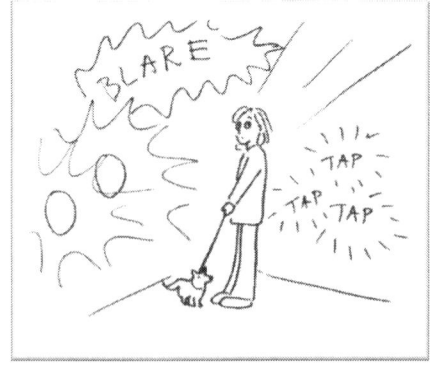

*to you. . . You should have known her car, but in the dark all you could see were the lights. The adrenaline had gone to work, because in spite of the fact that it's quite cold . . . there is a hint of perspiration on your upper lip. . . you did not recognize the car! Eventually you get back home . . . But you haven't achieved anything. Your shopping list is not planned, the outline for your conference report is not in shape. You had been too busy protecting yourself to get anything else done."*

Scary!

I hope this passage has given you some idea of just how distracting and disturbing such sensory distortions can be; how they can arouse great anxiety and also disrupt a person's" ability to think or act in a "normal" manner.

\*\*\*

## PRIMARY EFFECTS

**Anxiety.**

A major "side effect" of these problems is anxiety. Although not always obvious it is evident in:

- Obsessions/compulsions. These are integral to ASD and can include the repetitive (stereotyped) behaviors such as flicking a bit of string repetitively or lining toys up in rows and also the child's preoccupation with a particular subject so that he talks about one topic repetitively, or collects particular toys/items like dinosaurs. These are similar in effect to a young child's security blanket and, by giving him something to focus all his attention on, help keep his anxiety at bay.
- A dislike of change. This makes routine extremely important, providing some constants in a perplexing world. Reactions to change are very individual. Thus one child will become distressed by apparently small things, such as an item which is out of a place while ignoring larger changes whilst for another the converse is true.
- Withdrawal – as he tries to protect himself by ignoring or excluding anything which might provoke anxiety.

**Other Effects**

Anxiety will also limit his social interaction, the development of social skills and even his speech.

Similarly, it will interfere with his ability to concentrate, learn and/or remember things. He may also appear to lack curiosity simply because he is frightened of attempting anything new and this will inhibit his ability to explore and play. Children who do show curiosity often tend to direct it towards objects rather than people.

Prolonged stress – as happens when you live with such sensory problems day in and day out – can have several physical effects. Thus it:

- interferes with the digestive process and can cause severe stomach pains during or after meals.
- weakens the immune system
- leads to vitamin and mineral deficiencies.

Many such children - regardless of age or ability – also suffer from "panic attacks." These often result from acute anxiety, although they can also be caused by sensory or emotional overload or simply by too much direct attention.

They can lead to any one of the following reactions:

- He may become "frozen with fear" and be totally unable to do anything (even something nice like eating a cake).
- Fight or flight - he may suddenly: "attack" himself or another person.
- He may suddenly run away from a situation.

**Coping Strategies.**

The only way in which the child can make any sense of the world at all is to try and deal with the sensory information he receives a little at a time. In contrast to most people, who automatically process information from several senses simultaneously, this child can generally only process one piece of information at a time - "mono processing."

This is why he often uses peripheral vision (looking out of the corner of his eye or in quick short glances rather than directly at a person or object) as it helps limit the amount of stimulation he receives.

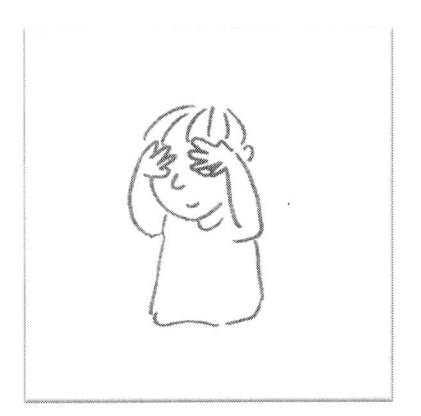

Mono processing also provides yet another reason for his slow responses. Taking in one piece of information at a times makes for a time lag between being asked a question and his reply – a delay that can make his answer apparently meaningless.

In some situations, the child may suffer from an information overload. For one child this might only happen in a busy holiday town or at a party with lots of people moving around and talking. For another an "apparently pleasurable" visit to the supermarket with its lights, movement, smells and noise, might have a similar effect.

The reactions to such overload are varied. One child may suddenly "explode" into hyperactivity while another might become more obsessive or compulsive as he attempts to contain his anxiety within manageable levels. Yet another might have a more severe reaction becoming extremely lethargic as his brain "shuts down" to protect him. When this happens suddenly this effect is sometimes mistaken for a form of epilepsy.

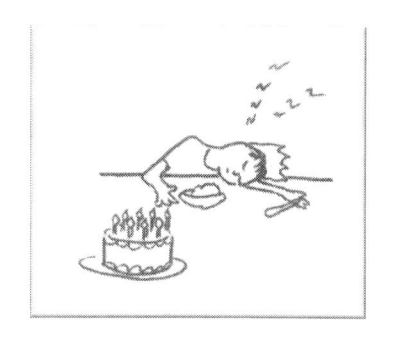

Some children have additional difficulties as, once the information reaches the brain, it is processed tangentially. For such children a single word or sentence can trigger numerous fast moving thoughts or images which, when verbalized, may seem random and unconnected to the matter at hand.

Thus an ordinary conversation about the holidays might begin with talk of a car journey and then move on to the destination and what happened after the person arrived. The child will be unable to follow this line of thought, as, at the very beginning of the conversation he may get stuck on the word "car." This will trigger a chain of thought about all the cars he has ever known; their shapes, sizes and colors. Indeed, he will probably still be thinking (and perhaps talking) about cars half an hour later, when the original conversation has long since moved on to other subjects.

\*\*\*

# E-FFECTS NOT DE-FECTS

**Learning Differences**

Unfortunately, the problems associated with abnormal sensory perceptions and anxiety also give rise to a whole range of cumulative effects. These effects, once again, range from mild to severe and vary from person to person. They will have a great impact on his life, interfering with his ability to develop relationships and learn. The problems do not affect everyone with ASD but can include:

- Poor short term memory. This can make life and learning extremely difficult. Such problems often coexist with a good long term memory (like that found in savants).
- Poor motor skills. These fall broadly into two groups.

    o Clumsiness; poor motor control; lack of coordination associated with the **gross motor skills** - e.g. cannot ride a bicycle - but can be very good at fine delicate tasks.
    o Problems using his thumb and doing **fine motor tasks** e.g. may hold his pencil in his fist. In contrast his gross motor skills may be good so that he may climb walls etc. and be seemingly fearless.

- Limited understanding of: directions, sequencing, sense of time.
- Mixed dominance. May use either hand to write, eat etc.

- Disorganization. Loses things; has difficulties organizing work etc.

In addition to the problems already mentioned the child may also:

- have poor self-esteem.
- have a poor or limited awareness of:

    o Danger - will not necessarily be as aware of danger as his peers. May not be able to respond in the correct manner to warning signs e.g. the noise of a fire alarm could cause him to panic or freeze rather than to leave the room.
    o Bodily functions - so that she may not realize that he needs the toilet until the need suddenly becomes urgent or it is too late.
    o Pain - unusual responses. May be very aware of pain. Alternatively, could ignore it - as with the boy who jumped up and down on a sprained ankle because he was upset at being taken to the casualty department!
    o Other peoples" motives - his inability to "read" faces and body language can make him seem naïve. It can also make him very vulnerable.

While some of his problems are obvious others will be subtler. His lack of awareness may cause him to:

- Seem offhand, self-centered or aloof.
- Make direct personal comments that can seem quite rude.

- Invade other people's personal space e.g. may stand too close to other people, stare at them or even touch items of their clothing.
- Become agitated or aggressive when frustrated or confused.
- Demonstrate age inappropriate behaviors e.g. laugh inappropriately, make odd noises, or have a panic attack (which is often mistaken for a tantrum).
- Have difficulty understanding social rules.
- Talk repetitively about one subject whilst missing the "clues" that indicate another person wants to speak.
- Have difficulties organizing or limiting his own behavior in an age-appropriate way.

**Please do not assume that he is being intentionally rude or negative or that the behavior is specifically aimed at you. Such behaviors are merely part of the problems.**

The problems detailed in this chapter and the previous ones can lead to great frustration and anxiety which, as already mentioned, give rise to withdrawal, stereotyped behaviors, a need for routine or disruptive behavior.

This risks becoming a vicious circle as any interruption to his preoccupations or change in "his" routine creates further stress. Generally, though these behaviors will decrease if the child feels secure and knows exactly what is expected of him.

Please remember that:

- Unusual behaviors (like having a tantrum in a noisy supermarket) do not necessarily equal naughtiness – although he may be naughty at times.
- An inability to speak does not mean he is unintelligent.
- He would if he could but all too often he simply can't.

**Vulnerability.**

His lack of awareness of others, visual problems and stereotyped behaviors often make the child stand out from his peers and, by drawing attention to his differences, can make him the butt of jokes or lead to bullying.

**Signs of Bullying.**

Bullying can take many forms from name-calling to social isolation or even physical violence, making life miserable and can cause a loss of self-esteem, depression or other mental health issues.

Sometimes, another child may encourage him to break rules or act in a strange manner, or "wind him up" so that he becomes agitated. Unfortunately, this bullying may not always be confined to children, for occasionally a member of staff will misinterpret ASD behaviors as "bad" behavior, and respond unhelpfully.

While physical signs such as torn clothes, cuts and bruises are easy to see the more subtle signs may be less easy to identify. Look out for changes in your child's behavior such as a reluctance to go to school, increased anxiety, wetting the bed, an increase in problem behaviors whilst at school.

Such changes can be the result of bullying but could have other causes too - such as a change of teacher, so you will need to liaise with the school in order to determine the cause/s.

**Communication**

It is also vital to find a way of helping your child to tell you of any problems. If he has difficulties communicating verbally, try using augmented or facilitated communication (also known as FC).

Alternatively, use puppets or toys displaying different expressions (sadness, aggression, etc.) to get him to describe what his day at school has been like.

**Cyberbullying**

While historically, bullying has been a largely school-oriented phenomenon, cyber-bullying and text-bullying is now on the increase. This allows bullies to torment, threaten, humiliate or embarrass their classmates via e-mail, instant messaging and through online communities such as Myspace and Facebook. The teenager who is able to use the Internet without support is obviously a possible prey to this awful form of bullying.

***Help protect him from such things:***

- Where possible get involved with your child's online activities.
- Know all the passwords and check them regularly.
- If your child has an online web page, such as with MySpace, visit it often to see what he or she is posting.
- Ask the school to suggest "reputable websites" that he can join.

**FOOD FOR THOUGHT**

Ongoing research indicates that many children with ASD suffer from one or more of a range of dietary/digestive problems which can affect the brain, behavior and mood.

The most common of these problems are:

- Food intolerances - especially to casein (milk) and/or gluten (wheat). The effects are generally Behavioural.
- Allergies to particular foods (e.g. chocolate, oranges etc.) which can cause hyperactivity or disruptive behavior – often within one or two hours of eating.
- Various other eating problems e.g. craves particular foods; eats non edible substances; has an excessive thirst.
- Reactive hypoglycemia (Low Blood Sugar Levels) This is generally associated with a high intake of sugar and/or junk foods and leads to a drop in blood sugar levels and a rise in adrenaline.
    They give rise to a variety of symptoms including hot and cold sweats, a loss of concentration, irritability, migraines or headaches; blurred vision, vertigo and/or a loss of co-ordination. The first sign is often a hot sweat (which may cause the child to loosen or take off her clothes). This may be followed by dizziness, trembling and, in severe cases, fainting.

Other symptoms sometimes occur including fatigue, nausea, headache, belching, poor appetite, backache, muscle pains or heartburn after eating etc.

A new bowel disease has also been discovered in some children in recent years. This can cause lumpy swellings in the intestine, recurring inflammation and constipation. While controversy now rages in several countries about the possibility of links between this bowel disease, "regressive" autism and/or the MMR vaccination it has to be noted that:

- this disease does actually exist (and can cause serious problems).
- treatment of the physical symptoms does cause the "autisms" to diminish.

This is particularly difficult area if the person is unable to communicate their pain and parents will need to watch carefully in order to identify the signs. These can be Behavioural as with one man who hid in a cupboard when he had toothache.

**NOTE** Many children with ASD also suffer from some type of epilepsy – a topic too large to feature here. For more information, please see resources at the end of the book.

***

## PARENT POWER

In the past a diagnosis of ASD (and most particularly of autism) was often linked to a doom and gloom prognosis. However, it is impossible to predict the future - or to accurately assess an individual's ability to progress – so such gloomy predictions should not be taken as fact.

They are not.

Even so living with someone who has ASD can be extremely difficult at times. This is not simply because of the child's behavior, but also because, even nowadays, you may still have to fight for some of the services your child needs.

Fortunately, though some help is available. This book should already have given you some insight into the reasons behind particular aspects of your child's behavior. This puts you in a position to make a real difference to your child's life, using a range of relatively simple ideas - which will generally make family life easier too.

Details of "stress-busters" and other useful ideas can be found in *A Survival Guide – Positive Parenting for Children with ASD.*

**DO REMEMBER TO TAKE CARE OF YOURSELF SO THAT YOU CAN TAKE CARE OF YOUR FAMILY.**

Getting overtired and overstressed can lead to illness and even possible resentment towards the child so it is vital that you find ways/times in which you can relax and make time to recharge your batteries.

This could include:

- A little "me" time - whether it be Listening to some music or watching a program that you enjoy or having a quiet cup of coffee or making an uninterrupted phone call.
- Time with your spouse – even if it is simply a dinner for two at home.
- Keep healthy. While most parents burn a tremendous amount of energy on a daily basis a short time exercising will give you a chance to get rid of tension and stress and benefit your health. That could include using exercise equipment to use at home or enrolling in an exercise class while he is at school – which will also introduce you to other parents.

***Potential Supports Include:***

- Your local autism support group, enabling you to share ideas and support.
- Libraries/toy libraries.
- Family and friends who can provide you with some 'space' on a regular basis, even if it is only a couple of hours a week.

NOTE: Your doctor should be able to offer advice and help you get further information and support. If not ask to see someone else. It may help to ask for an extended appointment and go armed with a list of questions/concerns.

**BOOKS**

Interesting autobiographies include:
A Real Person - Gunilla Gerland
Like Color to the Blind - Donna Williams
Lucy's Story: Autism and Other Adventures - Attwood & Blackman
The Reason I Jump: One Boy's Voice from the Silence of Autism - Naoki Higashida, David Mitchell and Keiko Yoshida
Carly's Voice - Arthur Fleischmann and Carly Fleischmann
Autism and Me - Rory Hoy
Beyond the Silence - Tito Rajarshi Mukhopadhyay
Born on a Blue Day - Daniel Tammet
Do You Understand Me? - Sofie Koborg Brosen
Emergence – labeled autistic - Temple Grandin
Life Behind Glass - Wendy Lawson
Living Through The Haze - Paul Issacs
Look Me in the Eye - John Elder Robison
Women From Another Planet? by Jean Mille
Books by Sarah Stup from http://www.sarahstup.com/


Other books include:
The Gift of Dyslexia - Ron Davis
Autism and the Myth of the Person Alone - Douglas Biklen & others
The Ultimate Stranger - Carl Delacato
A Teacher's Window into the Child's Mind - Sally Goddard Blythe
Reading by the Colors - Helen Irlen
Parents Guide to Vision In Autistic Spectrum Disorders - Ian Jordan
The Sound of a Miracle - Annabel Stehli

*\*\*\**

THE AUTHOR

Stella Waterhouse is a writer and therapist who has worked children and adults with autism and other learning differences since the late 1960s.

She was hooked . . . and has been ever since.

Stella wrote her first book on autism, Asperger's syndrome and other sensory disorders in 1990. The published author of several books including A Positive Approach to Autism, she has recently published Autism Decoded – The Cracks in the Code and is currently completing the second book in the series: Autism Decoded - The Ciphers.

*** 

If you found this book helpful, please leave a review. Many thanks.

**Meanwhile don't forget to claim your FREE gift**

**You can download it from:**
www.gerrysorrillpublishers.com

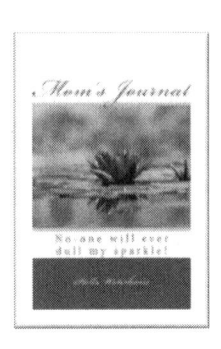

## Other FREEBIES re AUTISM

**Here are some FREE tools to help you on your journey.**

Grab the FREE checklist to help you identify whether your child has visual differences.

Have a child with auditory difficulties? Want to help? Get your FREE mini-course about the Auditory Differences and the Soundsrite Program.

Claim your FREE *Dietary Diary* here

Claim your FREE copy of *The Food Detectives Guide* here

**Go to: www.autismdecoded.com or use the QR code**

Printed in Great Britain
by Amazon